PERIMENOPAUSE

HOW TO CREATE A HEALTHY PHYSICAL & EMOTIONAL LIFE DURING THE CHANGE

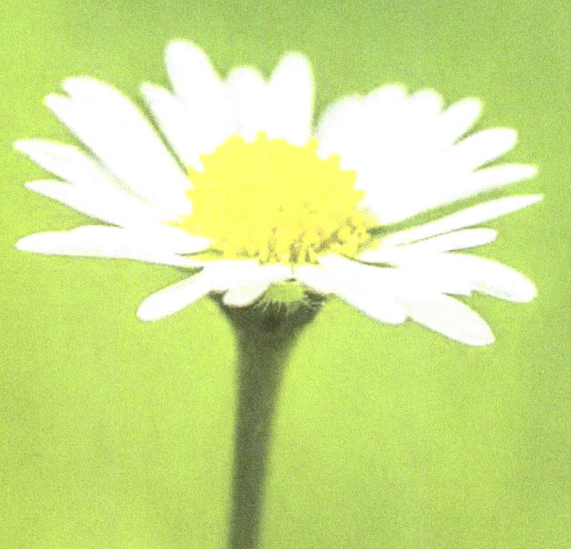

HEATHER ROSE

Perimenopause

How to Create a Healthy Physical & Emotional Life during the Change

Table of Contents

Introduction

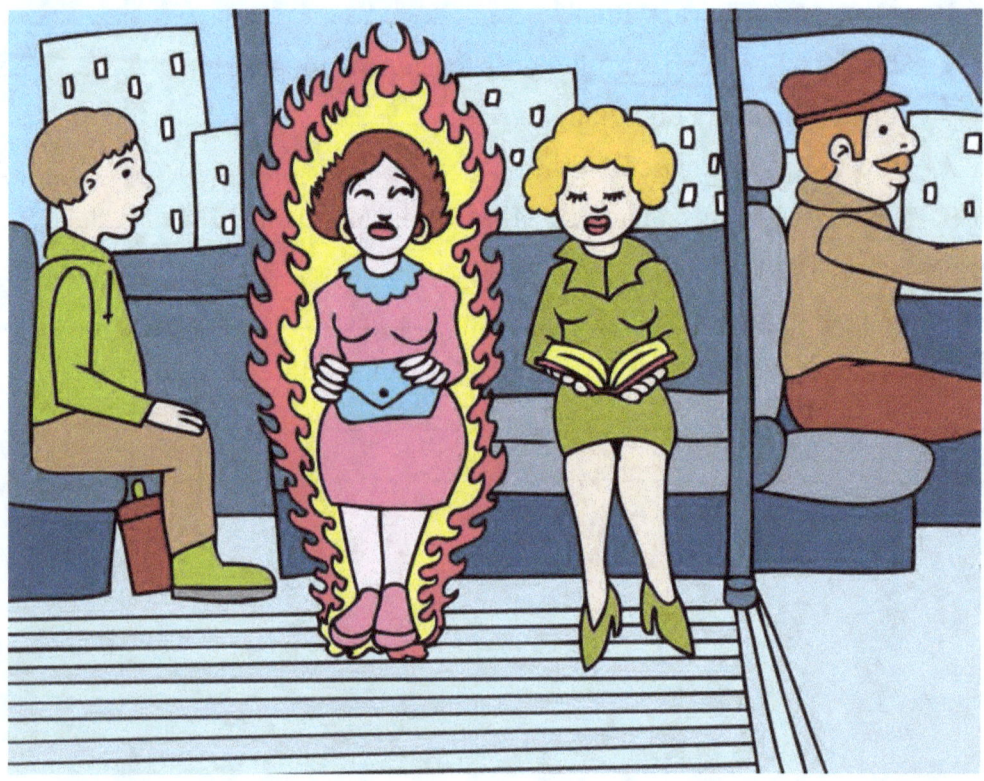

When you were younger, throwing a fit means you possibly experience PMS. You know you're getting older when other people refer to your mood changes as perimenopause.

Aaaaah. Perimenopause—one of women's most deterred words. It's quite understandable, though, as experiencing perimenopause will bring a lot of changes to a woman's body. Some women are lucky not to have those symptoms meddle with their lives, but some aren't so fortunate; their loved ones also have to adapt to the changes – especially about those mood swings – that they face.

The thing is perimenopause comes into a woman's life the same time as those other major changes. Midlife crisis, a marrying child, establishing careers... they all come at the same time, and why perimenopause chooses to interfere at these moments, nobody really knows.

What's necessary, though, is to learn more about this major change – understand what it's all about, what transformations will be taking place if any, how to ease the discomfort brought about by perimenopause, what foods can be eaten to alleviate the pain, which treatments can assist you with it – and understand what can be done about it.

Chapter 1 – What is Perimenopause?

Everybody is familiar with the term "menopause" and how it affects the life of a woman in general. However, there's another term that women have to be familiar about – it's called *perimenopause*.

Perimenopause – a Definition

Perimenopause, i.e. menopause or menopausal transition, is the stage that takes place several years prior to menopause. This period is when the ovaries slowly start to produce less estrogen.

The word "perimenopause" literally indicates the time "around" menopause. Medical providers use the term to denote the start of the estrogen decline, but women usually use this to imply the start of the exhibition of menopausal symptoms.

The younger the woman, the more worried and confused she may be as the symptoms exhibited by perimenopause differ for each woman, hence giving her confusion and anxiety.

Perimenopause Duration

Perimenopause starts at different ages. Progression signs are seen during a woman's 40s, but in some cases, the signs are seen during a woman's 30s, or maybe even earlier.

This stage lasts until menopause, when the ovaries finally stop releasing eggs. The estrogen decline should accelerate in the last one or two years of perimenopause.

The average length of perimenopause is usually four years. For some, though, this stage actually lasts only for a few months or as long as 10 years. Perimenopause officially ends when a woman is diagnosed with menopause – that is, a year or twelve consecutive months of not having her menstrual period.

Perimenopause Causes, Signs, and Symptoms

Your body responds as your ovaries change, and you start to produce less progesterone and estrogen as you pass the menopausal transition. The changes that take place during the stages of perimenopause are caused by the decrease in estrogen.

Perimenopause may be recognized when these signs and symptoms are being seen and felt:

- *Mood changes*. During perimenopause, irritability, mood swings, or an increased chance of depression can be experienced by women. This can be caused by various factors, two being hot flashes or other hormonal changes.

- *Sleep problems or hot flashes*. Hot flashes – that feeling of momentary warm sensation that comes with flushed faces as well as sweating – are quite common with perimenopause. The length, frequency, and intensity all vary. Sleep problems are caused usually by these hot flashes, but in some instances, these problems are experienced even without them.

- *Menstrual Irregularity*. During perimenopause, ovulation becomes more unpredictable. The length of time in between periods may become lengthier or shorter. Menstrual flow can either be light or heavy, and some periods may be skipped.

- *Decrease in Fertility*. The ability to conceive decreases as your ovulation becomes irregular. Pregnancy is still possible, though, as long as you are still having your periods. Birth control is still necessary if you don't wish to be pregnant – it's only no longer needed if you've had a full year of not having your periods.

- *Bladder and Vaginal Problems*. Vaginal tissues may lose elasticity and lubrication when the estrogen levels diminish. When you have low estrogen levels, you're also more prone to vaginal or urinary infections.

- *Sexual Function Changes*. Changes may take place towards a woman's sexual arousal and desire. However, if a woman has had adequate sexual intimacy prior to menopause, then this will highly continue through perimenopause and beyond.

- *Bone loss*. When estrogen levels decline, bones are lost more quickly than when they are replaced. This condition increases a woman's risk for osteoporosis, i.e. a disease that brings about fragile bones.

- *Cholesterol levels change*. Decreasing estrogen levels can bring unfavorable changes to the blood. Bad cholesterol – low-density lipoprotein (LDL) cholesterol –

may increase, and the good cholesterol – high-density lipoprotein (HDL) – may decrease as women age; both states bring higher risks for heart disease.

- *Other problems*. Some women complain of short-term memory problems as well as difficulty concentrating during the perimenopausal stage. Progesterone and estrogen play a major role in maintaining brain function, but not enough information has been gathered to distinguish the effects of aging and other psychosocial factors from those effects triggered by hormone changes.

Chapter 2 – You're Not Crazy. It's Just Perimenopause.

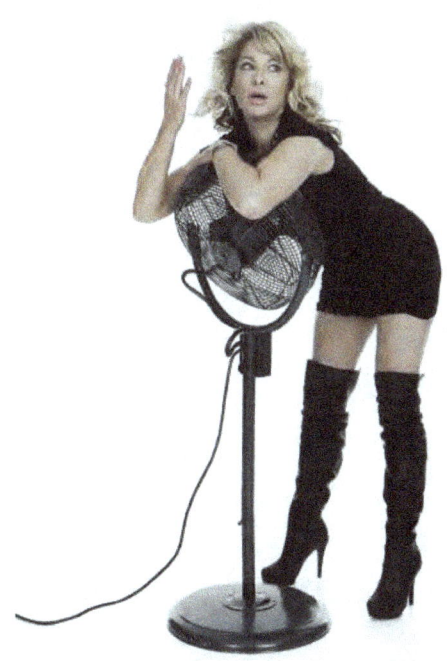

Perimenopause, down to the period of menopause itself, is a journey that becomes a struggle for a woman. Not only physical changes are encountered but also a battle of crazy emotions brought about by hormonal changes.

Don't worry, though. These changes are normal, and you can find workarounds for it. You're not crazy. It's not something you make up or something that's just in your head. You're just experiencing perimenopause.

A Woman's State of Mind

The period of time around menopause and a woman's mental health had a relationship that created controversies. There was even a psychiatric term for this – *involutional melancholia* – and this refers to the depression present in women that takes place when they undergo their menopausal years.

What makes this condition even worse?

Perimenopausal stress takes place around midlife, when a woman also undergoes other factors that add to the stress such as elderly parents getting sick, children leaving home due to independence, their spouse or they themselves experiencing health problems, and dealing with aging to name a few. These circumstances lead to women thinking more about stuff than they should, and this ends up triggering emotions that are not even necessary at times.

Mood Disorders

Women are known to experience a few of these mood disorders. The estrogen decline mainly triggers these mood changes, and these mentioned changes are eventually experienced by perimenopausal women.

Out of Proportion Anger

Women in perimenopause tend to overreact even to those little things. Responses may be viewed as "over the top" because perimenopausal women lean towards making a big deal about what others view as "small stuff." In response to minor events, women tend to be irritable and agitated.

Sleep Problems

Most perimenopausal women complain about sleep problems. During this transition to menopause, women are known to experience insomnia. Sleep problems are usually connected to changes related to age – sleep architecture, menopause symptom, or hormonal conditions – and according to research, women who are about to transition to menopause will have worse sleep problems than those who are on the pre-menopause stage.

Depression

Psychiatric problems are not common during menopause stages, but one out of five women is reportedly known to experience depression. Risks of depression are known to go higher during perimenopause and slowly go lower after menopause.

Panic Disorder

A panic disorder, the term used for unexpected and spontaneous occurrence of panic attacks, is quite common during perimenopause, and will exhibit more in women who showcase physical symptoms of menopause. Panic attacks are most prevalent on women experiencing perimenopause, and are associated with functional impairment, negative life events and medical comorbidity.

Bipolar Disorder

Women in perimenopause also tend to experience manic-depressive illness or more popularly known as bipolar disorder. If a perimenopausal woman already has bipolar disorder, then her symptoms and condition have great chances of getting worse. Women with bipolar conditions will also have higher chances of depressive episodes.

Obsessive-Compulsive Disorder

A woman during perimenopause may develop a case of Obsessive-Compulsive Disorder (OCD), have an OCD relapse, or have worse OCD exhibitions. OCD is defined by intrusive and distressing obsessive thoughts and/or recurring compulsive mental or physical acts. OCD fluctuations have been observed to correlate with menstrual cycles and with pregnancy, hence leading to ideas that hormone levels contribute to this condition.

Schizophrenia

Schizophrenia, a condition of the brain that affects a person's perception of his/her surroundings, can be seen in women approaching menopause. Observations lead to the theory that estrogen levels affect schizophrenia levels.

Chapter 3 – Physical Body Changes

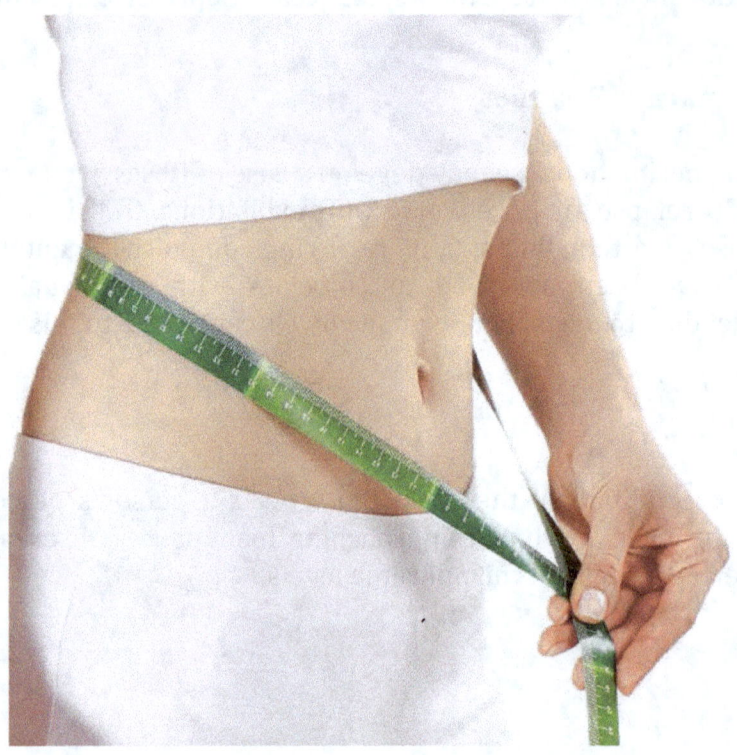

During perimenopause, changes take place – inside and out. Not only do you experience internal changes during this period – hormonal changes, to be more specific – you also experience physical body changes that will affect you.

As you approach menopause, how will your body change and adapt to this stage?

No Two Women are the Same

The perimenopause experience is different for every woman. Yes, there are chances that two women may undergo the same concerns, but that will be very rare.

The biggest differences are observed between women who have undergone natural menopause and those women with early or induced menopause who typically require dedicated care.

A woman who has experienced *natural menopause* states she doesn't experience any physical change at all, except the part where she experiences irregular menstrual periods that soon stop when she reaches menopause.

Perimenopause, or transition to menopause, is described by hormone changes. Women experience the signs at different times of their lives – no particular age, no particular trigger. A sign may be experienced or a woman may just be lucky not to have any bothersome indications of perimenopause.

Perimenopause = Sign of Aging

Why are women afraid of dealing with perimenopause (and with menopause itself)?

It's because it's a sign of aging.

When a woman reaches this point where she realizes she's about to reach menopause, she starts to feel dread and despair. It's when she starts to grasp the reality that she is no longer as young as she used to be.

This attitude is rather sad, but it truly happens to women, and it plays a major factor in the emotional disturbances experienced by them during this stage. Women who experience this include those who have delayed having children as well as those who still wonder if the conception of a child is still possible just before their biological clocks finally go off.

Women have been somehow "programmed" to think that their value lies within their capability to appear sexually endearing and to be endlessly supportive of men and to be nurturing and caring towards their children. Those traits are definitely good and of course positive, but on one end can be a one-sided argument as this won't help her develop her sense of self, hence her fear of aging.

Other Physical Signs of Perimenopause

Aside from the usual symptoms such as hot flashes, irregular periods, and mood changes, there are other signs of perimenopause – physical signs – that can be seen in a woman.

Acne

Because of changes in your hormone balance, your body may experience acne problems. What specifically triggers this is the drop in estrogen that could possibly lead to higher levels of testosterone and other male hormones i.e. androgens, hence, having acne as one side effect. The good news, however, is that once the menopause proper begins, perimenopausal acne almost always disappears.

Hair Changes

A small percentage of women reportedly experience hair thinning during and after their perimenopause periods. This is also related to high androgen levels that are no longer balanced by estrogen. About 50% of women experience hair loss or thinning before they reach age 50.

When the balance between androgen and estrogen levels shifts, excessive hair growth can also take place in various areas of the body such as the upper lip, chin, and cheeks.

Breast Tenderness

Another uncommon symptom of perimenopause is breast tenderness due to the body's changing estrogen levels. Sore breasts are a usual symptom of PMS, but this type of breast tenderness is more lingering and less acute.

During perimenopause, breasts become less dense as fatty tissues increase and glandular tissues decline. Mammograms become easier to interpret because of this.

Heart Palpitations

The reason behind this is unknown, but some women actually experience rapid, racing heartbeats during perimenopause. This is one of the more unusual symptoms of perimenopause, and yes, it can be quite frightening. It's reassuring, though, to know that it doesn't mean you are at risk for heart disease. It is simply a side effect of what your body is currently experiencing.

Chapter 4 – Is Hormone Therapy Ideal?

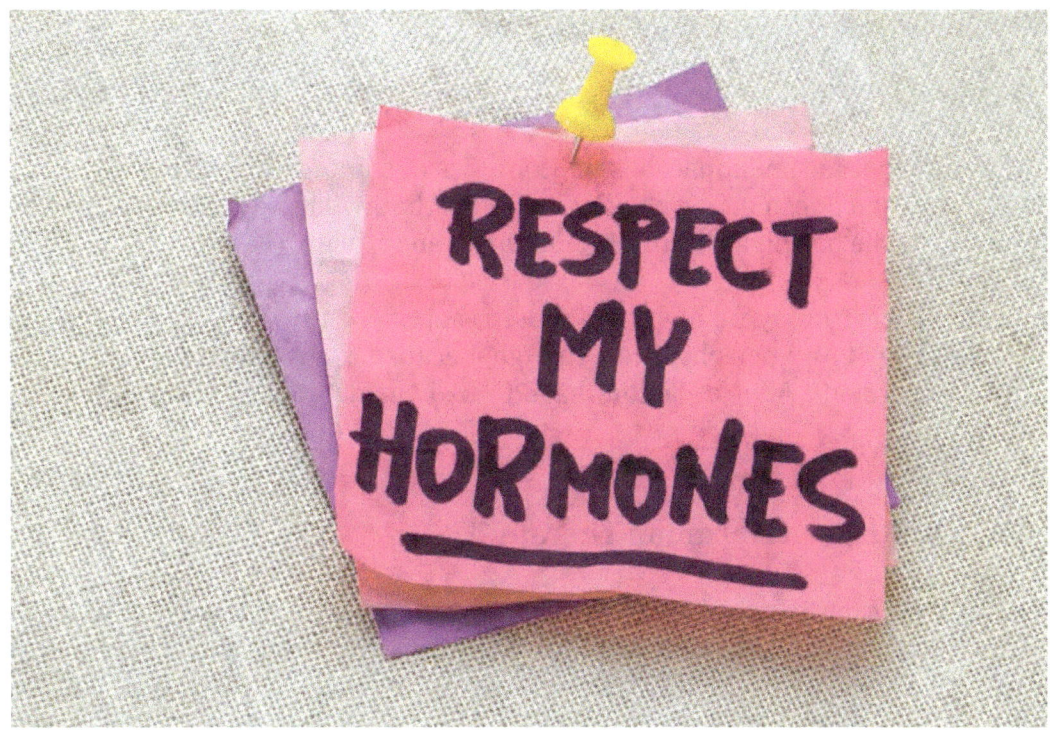

The hormone levels of a woman can be irregular and unpredictable during perimenopause. This condition makes her uncomfortable; her body works hard to adjust to the changes. Some women are lucky to not experience disruptions in their lives, but others feel discomfort which leads to disruptions in their daily lives.

That's why some women consider the option of hormone therapy when dealing with perimenopause.

What is Hormone Therapy?

Hormone therapy is a temporary treatment that aims to replenish a woman's hormones – mostly estrogen but may include progesterone levels as well – to help her gain the normal and ideal hormone balance. Hormone therapy is usually considered because it alleviates the symptoms of perimenopause.

Hormone therapy will be effective and least risky if the patient will be given the hormones with the lowest dose in the shortest possible time; the patient's condition will be monitored for six months.

When is Hormone Therapy Necessary?

The period of time that leads to menopause is a rollercoaster ride which is why some women tend to cross out options that will make the experience less bearable. Will all women be qualified for hormone therapy, though?

The following conditions, when met, will make a woman suitable for hormone therapy:

- If her perimenopausal symptoms are becoming unbearable
- If she doesn't have health conditions that will make her situation worse
- If she has high risk of developing osteoporosis

Hormone therapy may be a woman's last resort for getting relief. It should be agreed upon by the patient and her physician, though, because clearly, not everyone is eligible for this kind of treatment. A lot of factors have to be considered and a lot of risks have to be explained.

What are the Risks of Hormone Therapy?

Hormone therapy may help women pass the stages of menopause but as with other medicines and treatments, it's not risk-free. There are known health risks, and if you'd like to undergo hormone therapy, it's best to be aware of the other gambles you're going to take.

Blood Clots

Doctors are aware that estrogen intake will increase a person's risk of blood clotting. Risks are higher if the patient is also taking birth control pills that come with high dosages of estrogen. Risks will go even higher if the patient is a smoker. On the other hand, risks will be lower if estrogen skin patches will be used.

Cardiovascular Diseases

- *Stroke.* If a woman takes estrogen, she will have a higher risk of stroke.
- *Heart disease.* Estrogen can possibly increase the chances of heart disease in older women or those women who started using estrogen more than 10 years after they got their last period.

If a woman is known to smoke and has a heart disease, there are high chances she will be prohibited by her doctor from undergoing hormone therapy.

Cancer

- *Endometrial/Uterine Cancer.* A woman who takes estrogen therapy alone will have higher risks – more than five times greater – of endometrial cancer compared to those who don't. If progesterone is taken with estrogen, however, there will be protection against this cancer.
- *Breast Cancer.* There is a small increase of risk for women who have taken estrogen therapy for a longer duration. Guidelines indicate that hormone therapy is safe if taken within a span of 5 years.

Gallbladder Disease

Research shows that a woman who takes estrogen/progestin will have higher risks of developing gallstones. This is because high estrogen levels are connected to having gallbladder diseases.

Chapter 5 – Standard Food and Supplements for Perimenopause

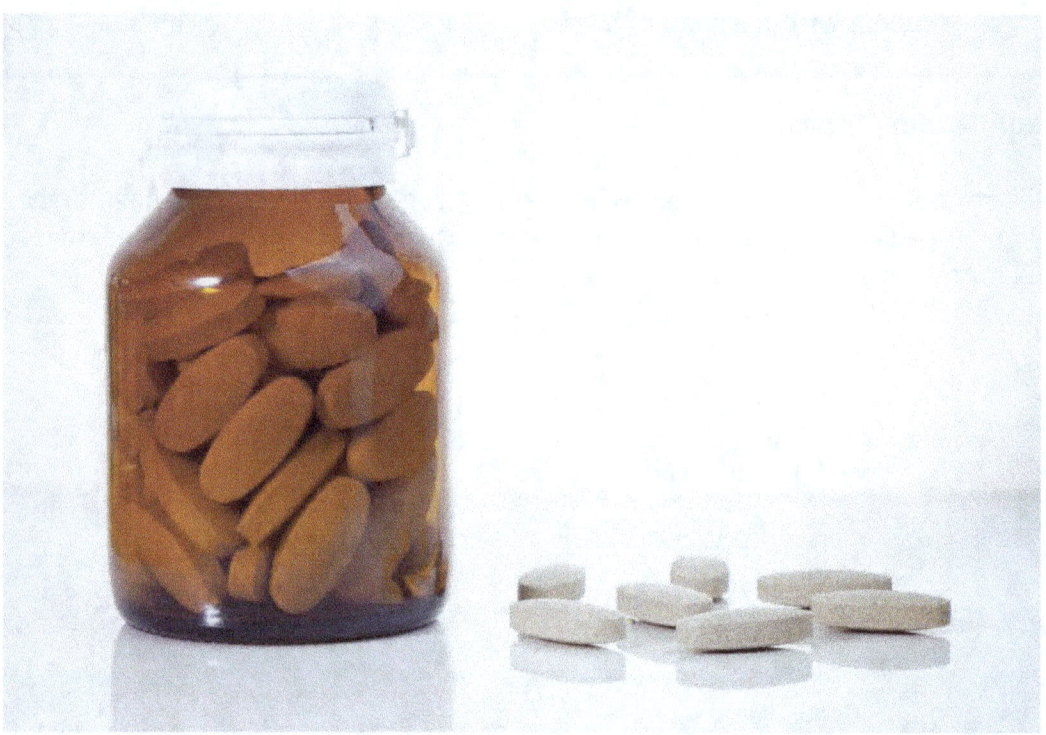

From hair loss to hot flashes to weight gain and weeping, perimenopause can be quite a discomfort to a woman's life because of hormone imbalances. A good balance can be brought about by taking the right vitamins as well as by watching your diet.

Natural Remedies for Perimenopause

Here are some natural remedies such as herbs that can help you properly manage your perimenopausal symptoms:

Flaxseed

Lignins, substances found in flaxseed, are essential modulators of hormone metabolism. Flaxseed oil is effective as hormone replacement therapy in alleviating sweating and hot flashes. This is also good for fatigue and depression.

Recommended dosage: Patients should take 1 or 2 tbsp. a day. Another option is to buy flaxseed that's ground up (or grind it yourself using a coffee grinder) and have it sprinkled on top of your food.

Evening Primrose Oil

Evening primrose oil helps in relieving anxiety, breast tenderness, irritability, mood swings, and headaches. It also helps in water retention. This is because it's a good source of gamma-linolenic acid that is an important fatty acid as it helps influence prostaglandin synthesis and also helps moderate menopausal symptoms.

Recommended dosage: Take 1000 mg each day two weeks before the start of your period. Take half of it during mornings and take half at night after dinner.

Soy Foods

Isoflavones found in soy foods can help you have some estrogenic activity and have balanced hormone levels. It can help decrease the intensity of night sweats and hot flashes. It can also improve your cholesterol and help lower your blood pressure.

Black Cohosh

Black cohosh is one of the best-studied and accepted traditional herbs for menopause. This herb is used to aid in decreasing symptoms of menopause such as hot flashes. What it does is to support and maintain a woman's hormonal levels, thus lessening the severity of hot flashes.

Recommended Vitamins for Perimenopause

Aside from foods, there are vitamins that perimenopausal women are advised to take.

Vitamin E

Having a daily dose of natural Vitamin E (400-1200 IU; 400 IU is enough once your hormones are balanced) can possibly help lessen symptoms of hot flashes. It can also help relieve mood changes, anxiety, insomnia, and tissue dryness. It also helps reduce risks of heart disease by preventing the bad cholesterol from sticking to the artery walls.

B Vitamins

The B vitamins, a group of water-soluble vitamins, can assist in making women deal with the stress brought about by perimenopausal symptoms. Your multivitamins must have around 50-100 mg of Vitamin B6 as the precursor to serotonin (the "happy" hormone).

Zinc

Zinc helps to decrease too much estrogen and increase a woman's progesterone levels. This also aids in building strong bones and in improving the immune system.

Recommended dosage: Zinc amounts should be around 15-50 mg each day.

Chapter 6 – Perimenopause Food Plan

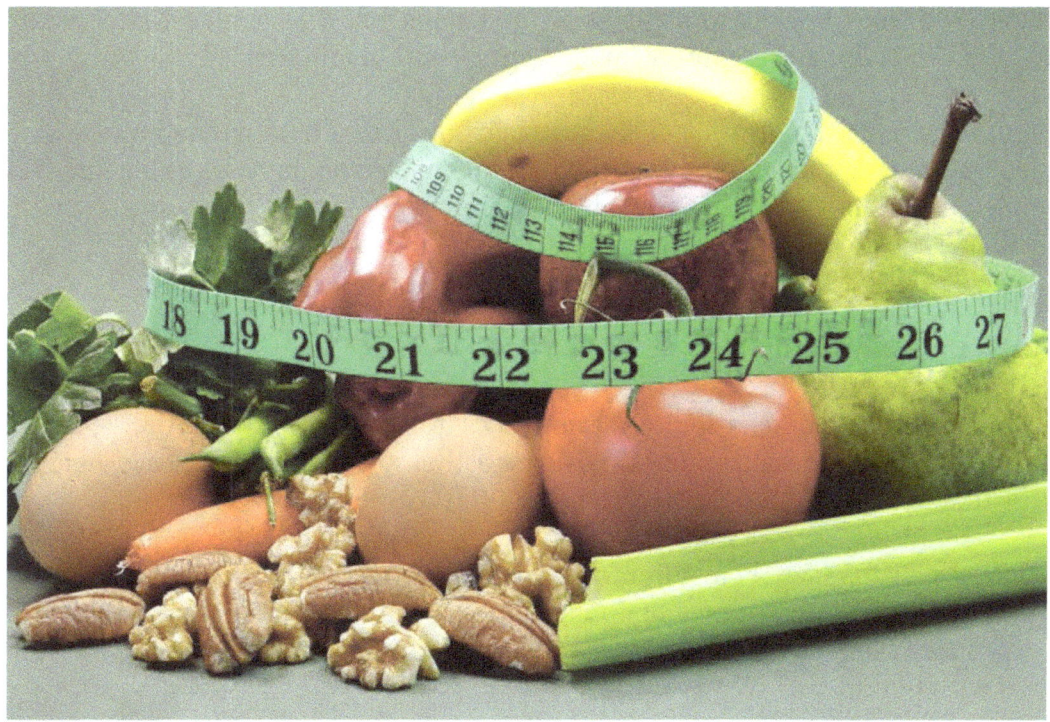

Your doctor will be your best ally in helping you manage your hormones, but it won't hurt to have a few dietary tactics that could keep you from going crazy due to perimenopause.

Eliminate the Big Three

For any hormonal changes, there are three things that make things worse: caffeine, sugar, and alcohol. These three compounds have the tendency to exaggerate any symptoms felt and can make things worse when stress adds up.

After eating foods packed with sugar, your blood sugar will also go nowhere but up. Having more than your necessary dose of caffeine will over-activate your "fight or flight" stress response, hence giving you more of that emotional roller coaster. Alcohol may be able to calm you down at the present moment, but then again, if you overdo it, it can have staying effects when you feel edgy the next day.

Have these three eliminated from your diet and you can see the results almost immediately.

Legume Load-Up

Women will gain several benefits from eating beans and lentils. This is because the combination of protein and high fiber helps to keep your blood sugar stable longer after you have had your snacks and meals – this helps provide a nice buffer against what perimenopausal women refer to as "mood swings within minutes."

Legumes also gain points for being low on calories that help women maintain a healthy body weight during those times that they are prone to gaining weight. Legumes also have B-complex vitamins – and that includes B6 and folate – that serve as enzyme cofactors involved in estrogen metabolism.

Stock up on Vitamin D

Perimenopausal women require Vitamin D as it helps in the absorption of calcium and it also aids in bone mineralization. Exposure to the sun's ultraviolet rays helps the body manufacture Vitamin D, and the body needs 200 IU each day.

Examples of foods rich in Vitamin D are salmon, cod liver oil, mackerel, beef liver, fortified milk, and eggs. If a perimenopausal woman lives in areas that don't have enough sun exposure, then she may need a supplementation for Vitamin D which should be checked with her doctor.

Crave for Calcium

Calcium is one of the best vitamins that a perimenopausal woman can take in. Calcium is the body's most abundant mineral. It is used for muscle contractions, secretion of hormones and enzymes, blood vessel contractions, and spreading of nerve impulses.

In a woman's body, majority of calcium is kept in the teeth and bones for structural support. As women grow older, the ability to form new bones declines, and this leads to osteoporosis and weaker bones.

A woman in the perimenopause stage will need 1,000 mg of calcium each day as confirmed by the Office of Dietary Supplements. It's best to include foods such as cheese, milk, yogurt, spinach, and fortified orange juice.

Omega-3 Fatty Acids

To have happy brain chemistry, you should get the right amounts of Omega-3 in your diet. Research has connected enough Omega-3 in a woman's diet to a better mood and less chances of depression. DHA, a main Omega-3 fat, is particularly loved by the brain.

To get adequate amounts of Omega-3, it's recommended to eat fatty fish – at least two servings – such as sardines, salmon, mackerel, tuna, bluefish, or barramundi weekly as these are nature's richest sources of Omega-3.

Add Some Soy

Certain research suggests that soy can help you stay cool when things get heated up, especially if it's supported by your family history.

Soy is good as it has phytoestrogens, naturally occurring plant compounds that have the ability to imitate the body's own estrogen. What it does is to bind with particular estrogen receptors that have the potential to help your body ease through the loss of your personal source of estrogen.

According to research, eating 2-3 servings of soy can possibly decrease the severity of hot flashes, protect you against heart disease, and reduce breast cancer risks.

Chapter 7 – How to Create Pelvic Health

During perimenopause, it's likely that your pelvic area isn't at its best condition. Particularly, the muscles in your pelvis stretching to the front and back sides of your body are undergoing pelvic floor prolapse. As a result, strength and stabilization are lost, and the vagina shifts to the bladder. In severe cases, gynecologists notice the presence of bulges around the vaginal area.

Here are some tips to create a good pelvic health:

Drink sufficient amounts of water

Water, as it is said, is a great treatment for almost anything, and this also includes pelvic floor complications. However, you shouldn't have glasses of the liquid excessively. For one thing, you'll end up urged by your bladder to race to the bathroom every 5 minutes or so. For another, you'll be constipated which won't be pleasant for your perimenopause problem.

No slumping and no straining

Especially if you're exhausted, it's an impulse not to be mindful of your posture. When you're tired, every part of your body is telling you to find the nearest bed to get a break. However, if you think slumping relieves you of fatigue, you're wrong. Not observing the proper posture when in a chair strains your abdominal muscles. Having unnecessary pressure exerted on your pelvic area isn't suggested. In fact, with this, you'll be experiencing more stress than ever.

Put on Kegel panties

The sound of simply wearing underwear while doing your pelvic health a favor seems enticing. Kegel Panties, introduced by a New Jersey urologist, are meant for strengthening the pelvic muscles due to the extensions sewn for the crotch. Having them on can be uncomfortable at first, but getting used to the feeling of wearing them can be accomplished in just a matter of days.

Remember that heavy lifting isn't for you.

If you have furniture to move or bags of groceries to carry, let someone do the job in your behalf. Conquering perimenopause will only be achievable and your pelvic floor will be as strong as it should be if you take it easy. If you think accommodating a load is considered a muscle-strengthening exercise, think again. It'll only make your condition worse, and being worn out is something you don't want to be burdened with.

Chapter 8 – Nurture the Mental Factors: Mind, Sleep, Mood and Memory

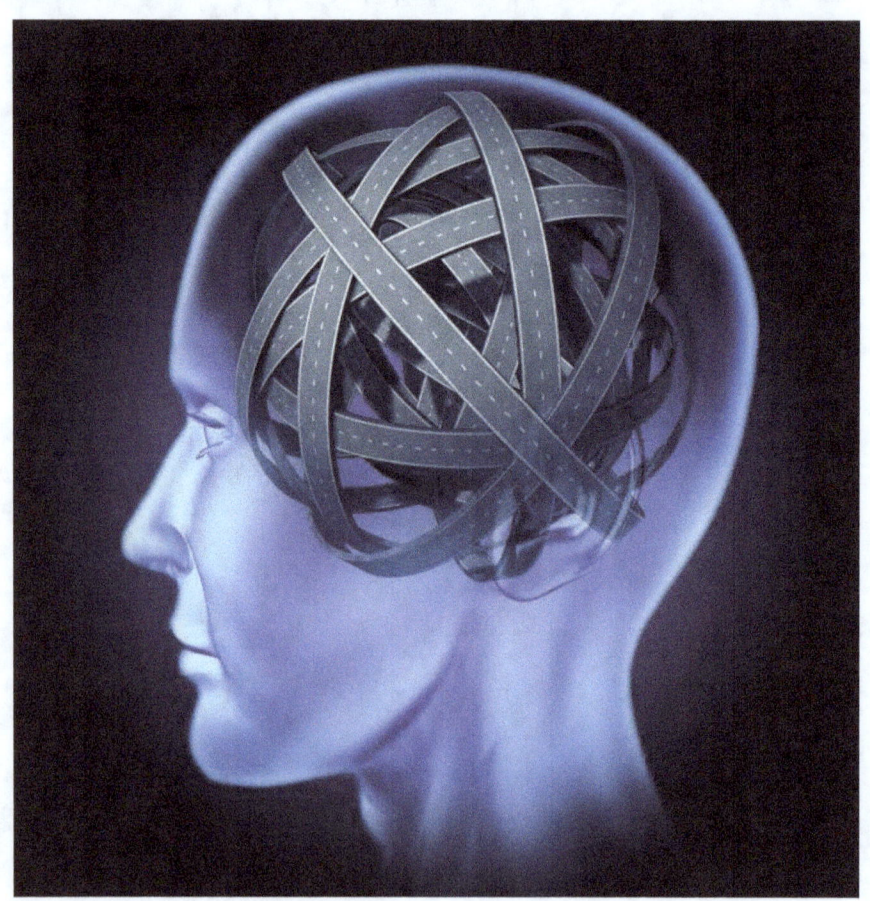

There are four mental factors that you have to nurture during perimenopause. These are your mind, your moods, your memory, and your amount – as well as quality – of sleep. These factors are somehow related, and if one of those mental aspects gets better, the other factors will also improve in time as well.

How do these mental factors help you as you go through perimenopause? How do you give them the nourishment they require?

Nurturing Your Mind

Estrogen levels are vital to your brain functions. Now, since this hormone level goes up and down during those periods of perimenopause, your memory, mental clarity, and thinking can suffer. Progesterone, on the other hand, can defend the brain against free radical damage as well as promote the repair of damaged nerve cells.

Your mind can be affected by stress. Stress can possibly worsen perimenopause symptoms, so it's essential to relax. So how do you take care of your mind and have it nourished? Here are some ways.

Get engaged in breathing techniques

Relaxation exercises can help you calm down during stressful moments. Breathing patterns are disrupted when you feel sudden emotions, and you can change them in a manner that helps you relax.

- *Deep breathing.* Visualize a spot just below the navel. Breathe into that particular spot and have your abdomen filled with air. From the abdomen up, let the air fill you, and slowly release it similar to deflating a balloon. Every exhalation should make you relaxed.
- *Rhythmic breathing.* Short and hurried breathing should be slowed down by taking long breaths. Inhale slowly first, and then exhale slowly. As you inhale, count slowly to five. Do the same as you exhale. Take note of how your body relaxes as you exhale slowly. Once you recognize the change, it will help you relax more.
- *Visualized breathing.* Look for a comfortable place where you can have your eyes closed and have your imagination combined with slow breathing. Imagine relaxation taking the place of tension in your body. Breathe deeply and visualize yourself taking in more relaxation.

Relax your mind

Aside from breathing techniques, guided imagery or mental imagery relaxation is a tried and tested form of relaxation that helps you establish harmony between your mind and your body. Mental imagery relaxation techniques help you create calm and peaceful images inside your mind – a form of mental escape.

Identifying your self-talk is important as well – understand what you say to yourself and how it affects you. Stay away from negative self-talk and always practice healthy and positive self-talk. Positive affirmations will counteract negative emotions and thoughts.

Getting Good Sleep

Having a good night's sleep will help your overall condition. With all the mood swings, night sweats, and hot flashes, a good night's sleep is still attainable.

When a women is about to reach menopause, she goes through a reduction in estrogen and progesterone. These hormones regulate sleep; hence, reduction of these hormones can lead to sleeping difficulties.

Try improving your habits if you have difficulty sleeping. If necessary, you have to ask your doctor for assistance. Medications may help you sleep better e.g. Benadryl – this can induce drowsiness.

Here are other good practices that can help bring about a good night's sleep:

- Exercise regularly. Take note, though, that exercise should be done at least 3 hours before your regular bedtime.
- Stay away from alcohol, caffeine, and nicotine. Reactions to these substances may differ from one person to another. Caffeine, for example, can affect your sleeping habits even if it's taken 12 hours prior to your bedtime.
- Have your thyroid checked by a blood test that measures hormones. Thyroid diseases are endocrine disorders that disturb sleep.
- Is stress keeping you awake? What you can do is to experiment with various relaxation techniques such as visualizing, medication, and deep breathing. You can also try to do the "body scan" where you become conscious of the stress and tension in every part of your body, and then you let the stress go.
- It all boils down to good sleep hygiene. Your bedroom should be kept dark and cool and it should only be used for sleep (and sex). Have a regular sleep schedule and stay away from heavy meals at night. Those reminders may seem obvious, but they preserve both the quality and quantity of your sleep.

Experiencing Good Vibes

Certain mood changes can be avoided by trying these tips – they reduce the impact of bothersome mood changes:

- Engage yourself in exercise. It promotes better sleep and in turn improves your mood.
- Perform mental stimulations from time to time such as solving puzzles or crosswords to sustain cognition and also to lessen chances of poor concentration as well as forgetfulness.
- Get involved in social activities so your mental function can be improved as well.
- If your symptoms are severe or if you need to handle stressful events, you can try seeing a counselor.
- Talking to trusted family members can also help.
- Maintain a journal or a diary that contains your feelings and your thoughts. By having this journal, you can keep track of identifying the trigger of your bad

moods. By doing so, you can think of strategies that will help you cope with such moods.

Memory Enhancers

Perimenopausal women have trouble with their memory. They also have difficulty in keeping themselves focused. This is because the memory capacity declines during perimenopause.

Certainly this is not noticeable and at times blamed on jam-packed schedules and hectic weeks, but the thing is you will be the main witness when memory decrease finally takes place.

What can be done to improve memory during perimenopause?

Play Games

Games – memory games, in particular – aren't just for kids. Research shows that mental exercise helps rewire and rebalance the brain. Puzzles hone your attention and processing skills as well as improve brainpower and make new brain connections.

Websites such as Happy Neuron, Luminosity, Posit Science, and CogniFit also give brain puzzles for better mental health.

Access Your Memory

Understand which mental tasks challenge your brain. Once you understand how those tasks work, utilize them to maximize the use of your brain.

Exercise

Working out is not only for the body but also for the brain. Exercise helps in the delivery of neurochemicals all throughout the brain to control and regulate the memory. Weight training, on the other hand, increases levels of the brain's growth factor that promotes growth, cell division, and health.

It's best to combine both strength and cardiovascular training to your workouts to get the highest benefits for your brain.

Have a Healthy Diet

Since your brain functions on food, it should then be fed right. According to research, people with diets that are high in Vitamins B, C, D, and E as well as omega-3 fatty acids have fewer chances of suffering from brain shrinkage and other irregularities connected to Alzheimer's disease.

A balanced diet has a major effect on how perimenopausal women act and feel. Food intake can either improve or worsen every perimenopausal symptom from night sweats to hot flashes to weight gains and mood swings.

Chapter 9 – Protecting Your Bones

It's not enough that you know how to give nourishment to yourself during the perimenopausal stage. You also have to know how to take care of the part of your body that holds you up – your bones.

In fact, it's not only during perimenopause that you'd learn to appreciate and take care of your bones; it should be done all the time regardless of how old you are. You should avoid cigarettes, eat well, and exercise regularly to give your body the TLC it deserves.

Perimenopause and Your Bones

As you reach this sensitive part of your life, there are additional things you have to do to make sure your bones will be strong all your life. Here are some ideal activities you can engage in for a better perimenopause experience.

Quit Smoking

This can't be emphasized enough. Women who smoke, compared to those who don't, have lower levels of estrogen and will reach menopause earlier – both of those lead to a lower bone density.

Watch your salt intake

If your sodium diet reaches an amount of more than 2,400 milligrams each day, it will lead to excess calcium excretion.

Have a bone-friendly diet and stick with it.

A bone-friendly diet is made up of fruits, vegetables, and dairy products that are low in fat. The ideal calcium consumption will be around 1,000 milligrams of calcium plus 400 to 800 IU of Vitamin D each day. Women in perimenopause as well as those who reached menopause should consume more than these amounts.

Move

Having a sedentary lifestyle is good, but it helps more if you exercise. In fact, according to recent research, exercising is better than high calcium consumptions and will have more impact on your bone strength. The more intense, the better. Lift weights, run, and jump rope – it'll do wonders for your bones.

Drink moderately

It's always a reminder to drink in moderation, and following that advice will lead to better bone health. Drinking moderately for women is equal to one alcoholic beverage in a day, and it's good for the bones as it can increase estrogen levels. Larger amounts will be possibly harmful, though.

Osteopenia vs. Osteoporosis

A low bone density can be two things: it can either be osteopenia or the more commonly heard osteoporosis.

- *Osteopenia* is the term used for the condition when you have low bone mass, but not low enough to be osteoporosis. According to research, one out of five women on perimenopause has osteopenia.
- Osteoporosis is the more serious condition wherein your bones have lost a major amount of density that they are already more prone to fractures, more particularly in parts such as the spine, hips, and wrists. Bones will be more porous when they are in this condition. Osteoporosis can occur in any age but is more common during the stages of menopause.

Other Tips for Better Bones

Perimenopause takes place more often in your 40s. What can be done to better prepare for menopause?

Assess your risk factors for osteoporosis. Be careful if you meet the following risks:

- if you've experienced fractures as an adult
- if you have a history of fractures or osteoporosis in your family
- if you smoke
- if you're thin
- if you've experienced having an eating disorder
- if signs of menopause manifest prior to reaching age 40

If you've met the previous "criteria," then you should be more careful as you have a higher risk of having osteoporosis. If you're around the perimenopause stage, discuss this with your doctor to have your bone density measured.

Keep an eye out for and be aware of missed periods. If you're entering your 40s and you're starting to skip periods, you might be entering the perimenopausal stage. This means it's time to step up on your plans for protecting your bones. Perhaps you'd need more strength training exercises or maybe take more calcium supplements. Doctors say that when your periods start becoming irregular, that's also when the bone mass decline begins.

Chapter 10 – Engaging in Your Breast's Health

As years pass, you learn to take care of your body more. Along with the other parts of your body, your breasts need your care and attention.

Some women tend to be not satisfied with their breasts – they may find these too big, too small, or maybe not as youthful and firm as what these once were. However, all women may agree that all they want is to have healthy breasts their whole life.

As a woman grows older, particularly as she reaches her 30s, 40s, or 50s, her breasts change as well. During the childbearing years, her concern may be about breastfeeding affecting her figure. During menopause and beyond, though, her main concern may be about avoiding breast cancer.

How can a woman take care of her breasts during perimenopause?

Breast Care during Perimenopause

Mastalgia, or breast pain, is not simple. There's no particular cure. It's a pain that can't be ignored; in fact, it even causes sleepless nights.

If you're experiencing breast pain, you might consider various alternative and conventional medicines to receive relief.

Do the Basics

Don't overlook the basics. Talk to your health care provider about the processes necessary. If you're 35 years old and above, you should consider undergoing a mammogram. It may not be sensible yet to have one, but it's best to undergo the process while your breasts are least tender.

An ultrasound may be necessary if you've had a mammogram or if you're under 35. Cysts can be revealed by an ultrasound – it's important to know if you have these cysts because you don't feel them but they expand and stretch your nerve fibers, hence causing pain. Sometimes, simply knowing that your lumps are benign, or your ultrasound gives you normal tissues as a result, is very reassuring.

Breathe

The swelling, breast pain, and sensitivity you feel are usually related to hormonal imbalances. Hormones are usually going crazy when a woman reaches her 40s.

Breast pains usually mean you have excess estrogen which follows your menstrual cycle. What you can do to keep track of this is to have a calendar, even just for a few weeks, and see if a pattern can be located.

Having gentle phytotherapy can possibly aid in maintaining the balance between your estrogen and progesterone levels, and by taking high-quality vitamins and minerals that have omega-3, you can help give your body the tools it requires to maintain a proper balance.

Try a massage

If there is a trigger point, you can try to massage the area yourself. You can also find a specialist for lymphatic massage. Usually, the problematic area is the breast's upper outer part where an underwire point hits.

Check Your Diet

Unfortunately, there's no proven diet that triggers breast pain for women, nor a diet that will cure it for everyone. Caffeine, though, has been known to affect women because it stretches nerves and dilates vessels, and once these women cut back on coffee, they almost immediately find relief. For other women, salt works the same way.

Excess estrogen can be flushed out by increasing the intake of fiber and green leafy vegetables.

Take Care of Yourself

Sometimes, all you need to do is to take a break and let yourself rest for a little while. Stress could be a reason why breast pain and menopause are related.

Do what you wish to do. Relax. Do something just for yourself.

You don't have to worry; a small percentage of women will still feel breast pain during their 70s, but for most women, most of the breast pain experienced goes away after menopause. Hormones are still a puzzling matter for some – you are all the same yet very different. However, all you need to understand is that it's all pretty normal; it's just that not everybody has the same symptoms.

Chapter 11 – Dealing with your Mind and Body during Midlife

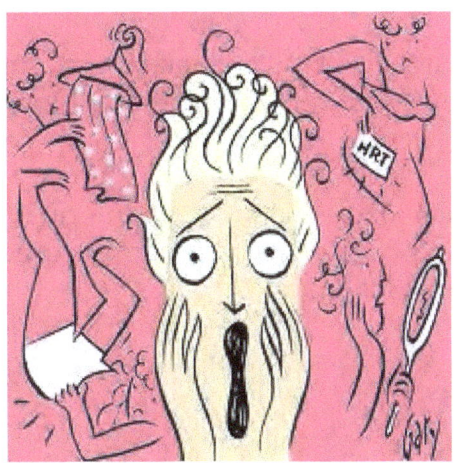

You've reached your 40s. You're irritable, moody, and easily agitated about everything. Don't worry; nothing's wrong. You've arrived at the perimenopausal stage during the middle ages of your life.

You may have thought you've gone crazy. No, an alien force did not take over your body. Perhaps you're unhappy about entering perimenopause. Maybe you're at that point where you're wondering where you are, what you've attained, and whether or not you can start over.

You're not alone.

It's not only the physical changes that bring suffering. The emotional changes make women puzzled as well, and it can lead to heartfelt and important questions. The answers aren't always welcomed, though. The answers could be upsetting as women often think of going back to their pre-menopause selves.

Regardless of what perimenopausal women think, they'd feel as if they're in a fullblown midlife crisis.

Midlife

People usually call midlife "the prime of life," and upon observation, you'll see that it really is.

During midlife, you're most likely healthy and productive. You have set goals and you have plans on where to go next on your life. Midlife is a busy time and it's sprinkled with changes. Perhaps you change careers. You go back to school. You get engaged in new hobbies.

Perimenopause and Midlife

Perimenopause is a natural event. As previously mentioned, same changes take place in every woman, but they cope and adjust differently. Women don't experience the same symptoms at the same time.

It's best to face perimenopause with a well-informed mind and a sound body. By knowing what to expect and by being physically prepared for it, you can take steps to prevent problems and ease symptoms.

Feels Like a Midlife Crisis

Experiencing perimenopause doesn't have to feel like you're in a midlife crisis. The manner you deal with it depends on how you view it.

It's your choice: you can see midlife as a time to panic, or you can look at it as a time for transition, a time for your personal growth.

Why does perimenopause feel like a midlife crisis? It's because media focuses on women's youth, perfection, and beauty. Hence perimenopause and its changes are viewed as a crisis. Furthermore, perimenopause changes contribute to depressive episodes.

When perimenopause – and eventually, menopause – finally sets in, you could feel a little off balance. It feels like you don't deal with a full deck. At times you're confused and you don't know what's going on.

Perimenopause doesn't always have to be put in a bad light. It can be seen as a positive thing – after all, this comes with happy changes: you no longer deal with raising kids. You no longer have to worry about preventing pregnancy. You can enjoy life. Won't these feel liberating?

Chapter 12 – Using Hormone Balances

Each hormone is responsible for completing tasks in the body. Understanding what every hormone does will help you determine which hormone is lacking and which hormone levels have exceeded.

Here are the types of hormones:

- Estrogen – The primary sex hormone for women. This speeds up metabolism, reduces muscle mass, increases fat stores, helps in forming secondary sex characteristics, promotes the uterus' increased growth and formation, and increases sex drive.
- Testosterone – It may be the main male sex hormone but it's still present in women. It contributes to a woman's libido and is responsible for the changes that women experience during puberty such as changes to the vocal range, acne, and growth cycle completion.
- Progesterone – Usually known as the "pregnancy" hormone, progesterone prepares the uterus for accepting a pregnancy. When progesterone decreases, this helps in labor and in milk production.

- Prolactin – This is the main hormone responsible for mammary glands' stimulation for triggering lactation. This also helps in the development of the fetus inside the mother's womb during pregnancy and is responsible for counteracting and concluding arousal.

Hormone replacement therapy, for the past few years, has become one of the most heated and highly debated topics. A lot of women are looking for better and more natural alternatives to take the place of "standard" hormone therapy.

Because of perimenopause, women experience difficulty triggered by varying cycles of progesterone and estrogen. These difficulties include night sweats, hot flashes, weight gain, and mood changes. These events can go on for years and it may take a while before they go down to post-menopausal levels.

How do you balance your hormones?

- If you can't avoid caffeine, you can at least minimize your intake of it. Too much caffeine can bring chaos to your endocrine system, more so if there are other factors involved that stress your hormones such as presence of toxins, pregnancy, beneficial fat imbalance, and/or stress. You can also replace coffee with herbal teas.

- Steer clear of fats regardless if it's peanut oil, vegetable oil, Canola Oil, soybean oil, shortening, margarine, or any other chemically altered fats. If you're going to integrate fats in your diet, it has to be one of the following: real butter, coconut oil, olive oil, and other types of animal fats. Eating lots of fish is recommended, especially if these are high in Omega-3.

- Fill up on minerals. Most women are deprived of minerals. They get depleted by phytic acid in whole grains. Minerals are also a major part of the body, and are essential nutrients of the body as well.

- Consider herbal remedies. They have been proven helpful for both physical and psychological symptoms. You have to consider and talk to a trained practitioner first before you completely use the herbal remedies as its effects may differ from one person to another.

- Eat foods dense in nutrients. Eat balanced meals; make sure you have plenty of fish, meat, good fats, bone broth, fruits, and vegetables in your diet. Some of the most nutritious foods are organ meats (e.g. heart, liver, kidney) and shellfish (e.g. oysters, crabs, clams, shrimp, and mussels).

Conclusion

You had puberty when you were younger. You were able to survive it. Now you have perimenopause that makes you find a new direction in life. For sure, you'll be able to survive it as well.

During perimenopause, your priorities change. From creating and nurturing your own family and career, your main concern is now about nurturing yourself.

It's just a stage – the hormonal shifts you experience will eventually settle down, and the mood swings will soon stabilize. After you get through this, you'll renew energy to pursue whatever dreams you have for your life.

Yes, outward appearances will change, but life and aging will bring a new woman out of you. From your past experiences to your desires and dreams for the coming years, you have a new life waiting for you.

Instead of wallowing in the negatives of perimenopause, it's best to think of all the dreams that are ready to be fulfilled. You think you ran out of time? Not really, as time is still on your side. Your life is waiting for you to conquer it completely.